The Princess and the Ruby

An Autism Fairy Tale

✳✳✳

By Jewel Kats

Illustrated by Richa Kinra Arts

From the Fairy Ability Tales Series
LOVING HEALING PRESS

The Princess and the Ruby: An Autism Fairy Tale
Copyright © 2012 by Jewel Kats. All Rights Reserved.
Illustrated by Richa Kinra Arts
Edited by Tyler R. Tichelaar
From the Fairy Ability Tales Series

Library of Congress Cataloging-in-Publication Data

Kats, Jewel, 1978-
The princess and the ruby : an autism fairy tale / by Jewel Kats ; Illustrated by Richa Kinra Arts.
pages cm -- (Growing with love series)
Audience: 6-8.
Audience: Grades K to 3.
ISBN 978-1-61599-175-4 (pbk. : alk. paper) -- ISBN 978-1-61599-176-1 (ebook)
1. Autism--Juvenile literature. 2. Autistic children--Juvenile literature. 3. Princesses--Juvenile
literature. I. Kinra, Richa, illustrator. II. Title.
RC553.A88K39 2013
618.92'85882--dc23
2012036159

Learn more at www.JewelKats.com

Published by:
Loving Healing Press
5145 Pontiac Trail
Ann Arbor, MI 48105

www.LHPress.com
info@LHPress.com
Tollfree (USA/CAN) 888-761-6268
Fax 734-663-6861

Distributed by: Ingram Book Group (USA/CAN), New Leaf Distributing (USA),
Bertram's Books (UK), Agapea (SP), Hachette Livre (FR)

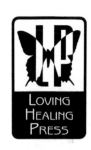

FOR EVERY PARENT OR GUARDIAN OF A CHILD WITH AUTISM SPECTRUM DISORDER.

The silver moon glared down at the old kingdom below. Snow blasted without a hint of mercy. Cold, gusting wind had knocked down tall ice-lined trees.

But nobody could have predicted what would happen next...

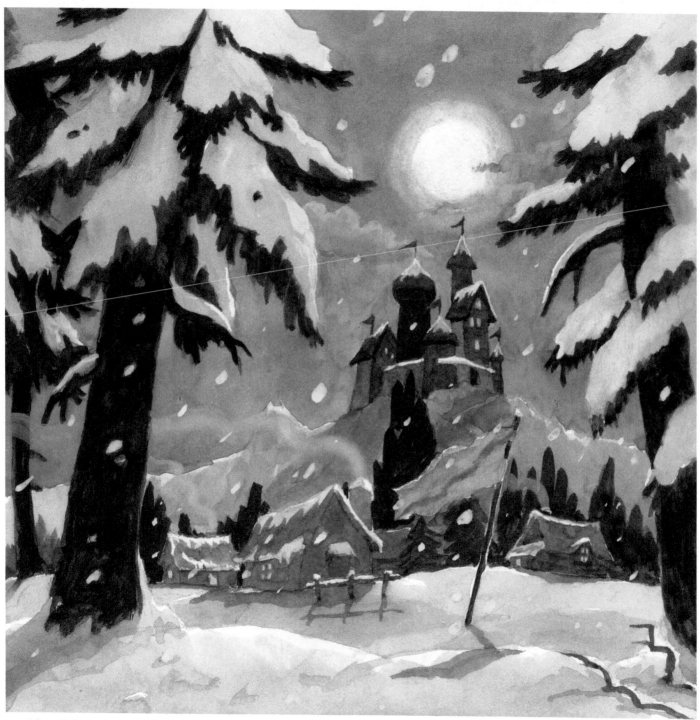

The Princess and the Ruby

Five loud chimes sounded at the gateway to the castle of the king and new queen. Somebody had arrived in the dead of night.

"Who in the world could that be?" the king asked.

Together, he and the queen made their way to the front entrance in record speed.

Worry that something had happened in the kingdom hung over their dampened thoughts.

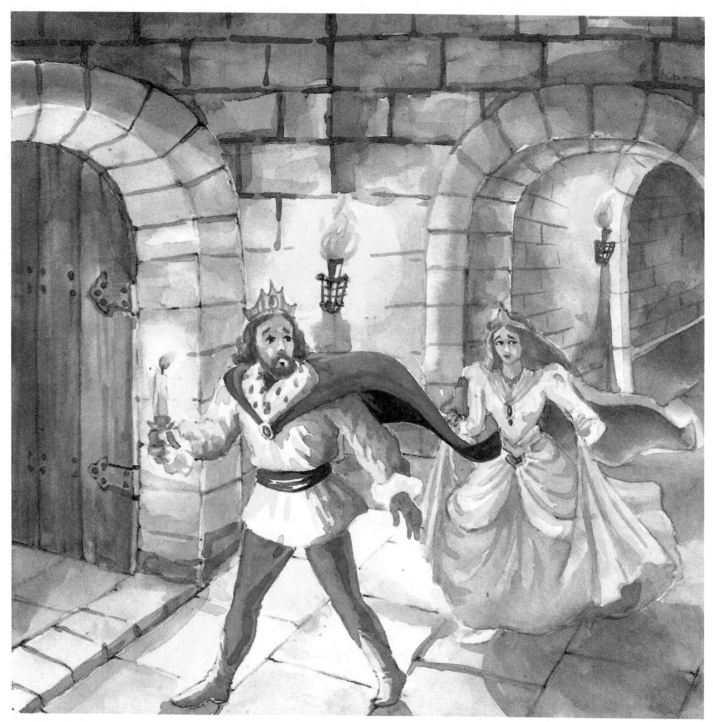

The Princess and the Ruby

When they arrived, the palace butler had already unlocked the door. He appeared dumbfounded at what he saw.

In the castle entrance, a young girl—no more than eight-years-old—stood shivering in a dark purple jacket. Her hands clung to a small black pouch.

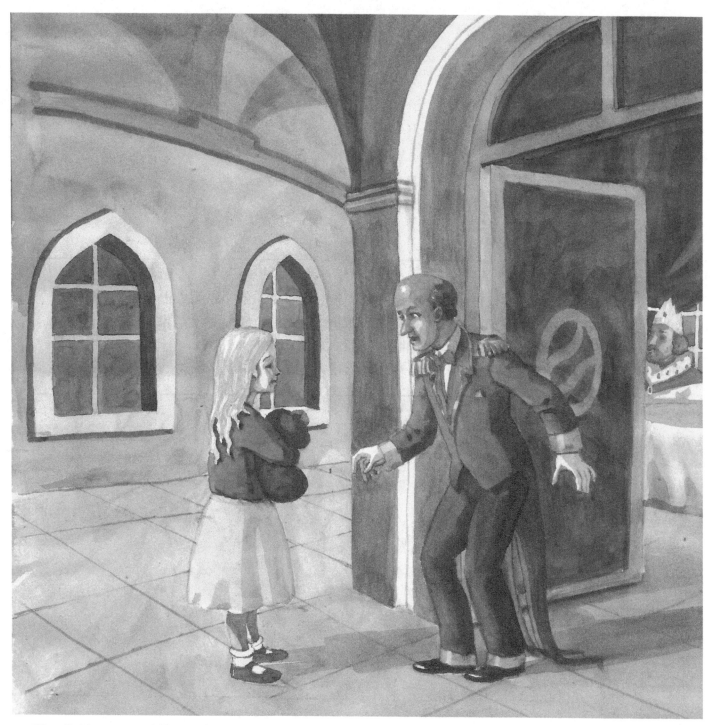

The Princess and the Ruby

Warm tears of joy sprung from the king's eyes. He looked up silently in blissful prayer, not believing his good fortune. Then he spoke. "Child, you've finally come back to me!"

But the young girl stared at him blankly. Words failed to escape from her dry, chapped lips. Instead, she began to spin in circles.

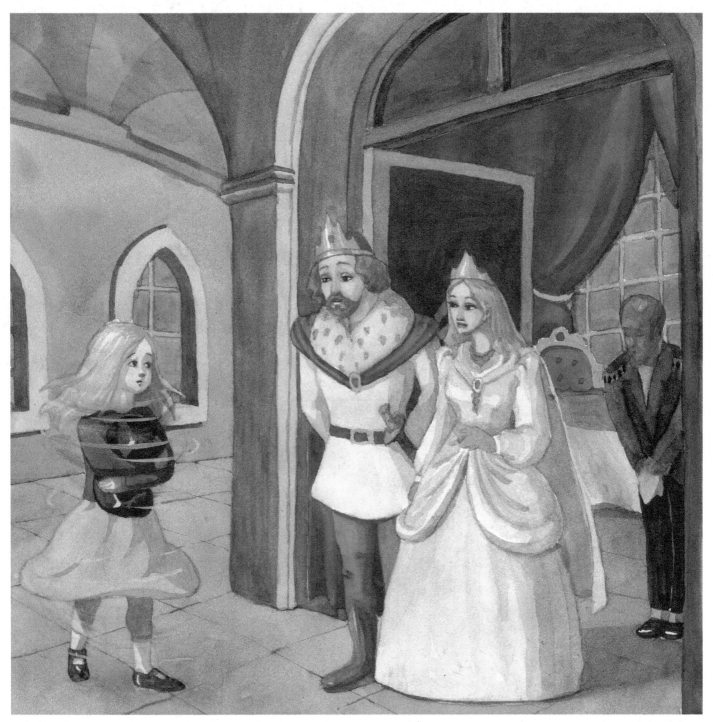

The Princess and the Ruby

The new queen burst out in laughter. "There is no way this—this wild being—can be the long lost princess."

"Hush!" the king exclaimed. "She has her mother's eyes. Poor woman died before her time."

The king gently took the little girl by her arm. "You must be awfully hungry."

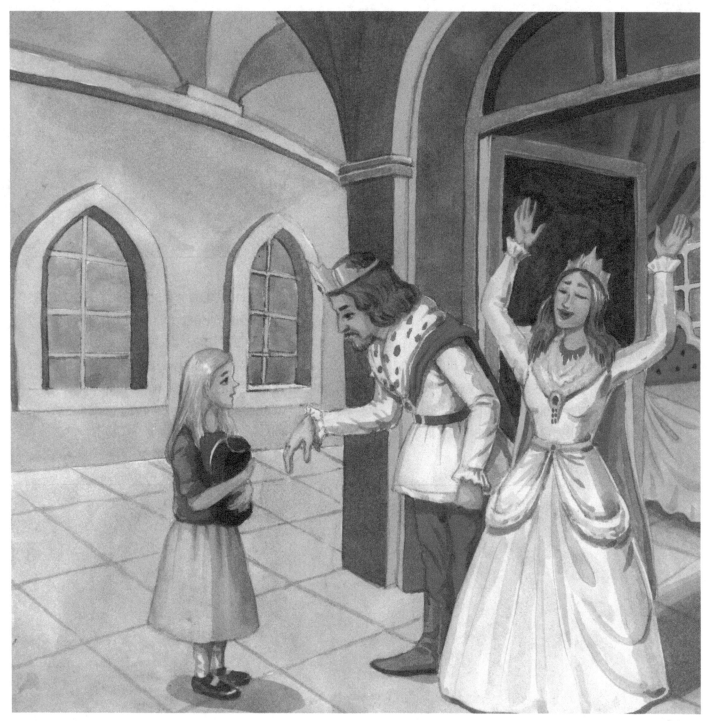

The Princess and the Ruby

The royal couple and the little girl sat down to dinner at their dining table.

The little girl was unaffected by the lavish settings. Rather, she opened her beloved velvet pouch, and from it, she dug out rocks of no bank value. Carefully, she lined them up in front of her plate. Then she began to sway back-and-forth in her chair in a most peculiar fashion.

The new queen looked on with disgust. "A real princess would have polished manners. She would never, ever play with some ugly, valueless rocks."

The king raised his palm. "The girl's rock collection is beautiful; just as she is. These rocks belong to the earth, and so does she. I'm a lucky man to be her father."

His wife gritted her sharp teeth.

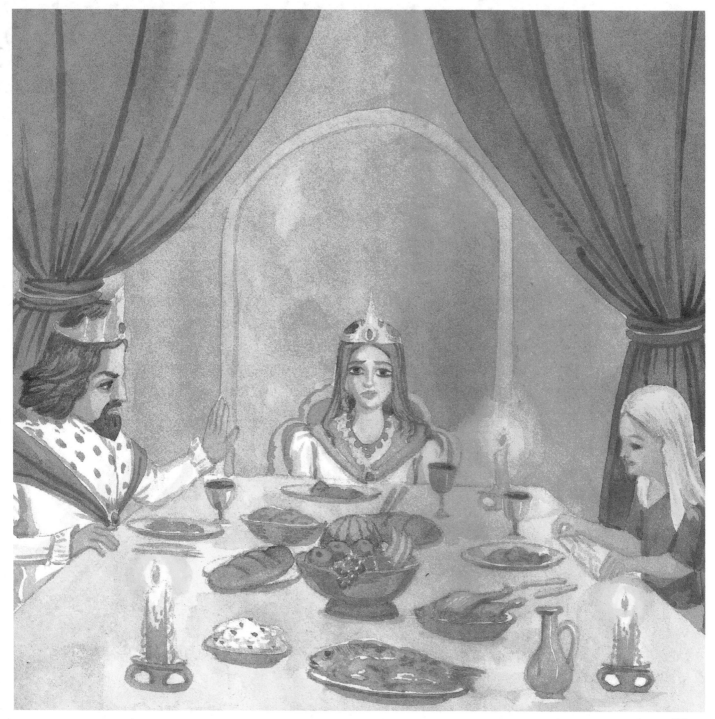

After their meal, the king ensured the little girl was given the finest set of silk pajamas.

Meanwhile, the new queen paced in front of the palace's secret jewelry lock box. A devious plan ate at her brain. *I must prove to the king that the girl is NOT his missing daughter. She's a good-for-nothing nobody! If she were of real royal blood, she'd only play with precious items.*

With shaking hands, she unlocked the kingdom's most prized gemstone. . . a huge, breathtaking ruby.

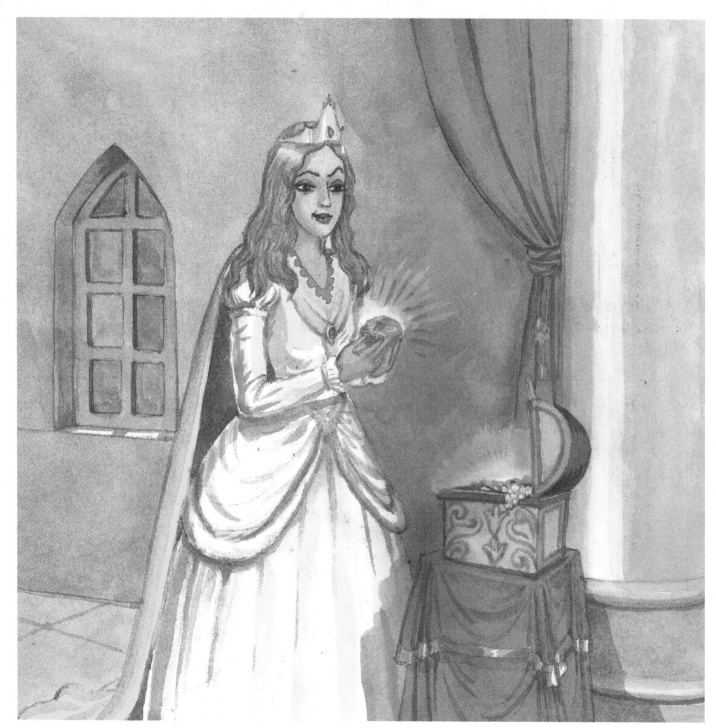

The Princess and the Ruby

With the help of the royal butler, the new queen prepared the guest room. In total, twelve bed mattresses were stacked one on top of another.

The new queen looked at her butler. "I can take it from here."

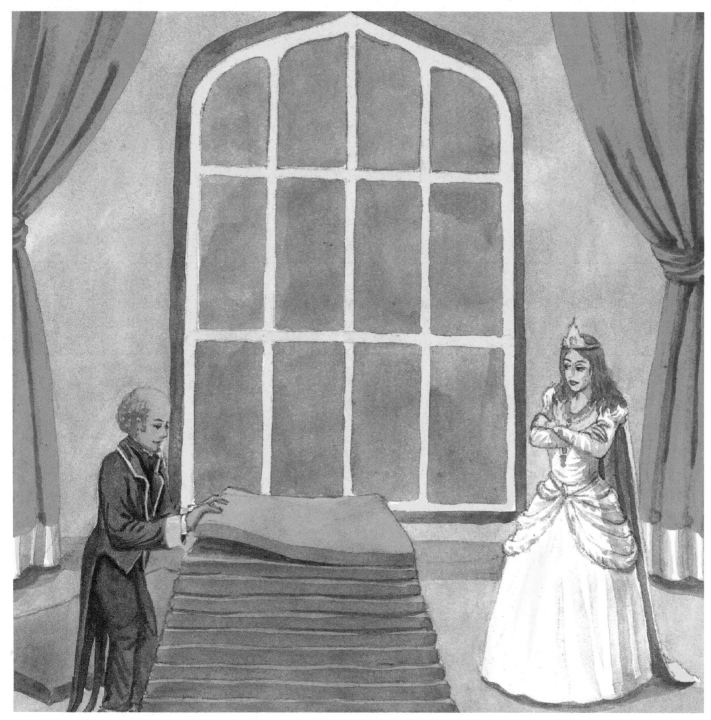

The Princess and the Ruby

Once alone, the new queen placed the kingdom's prized ruby in the center of the mattresses. "Let's see if this *supposed* missing princess feels this," she scoffed.

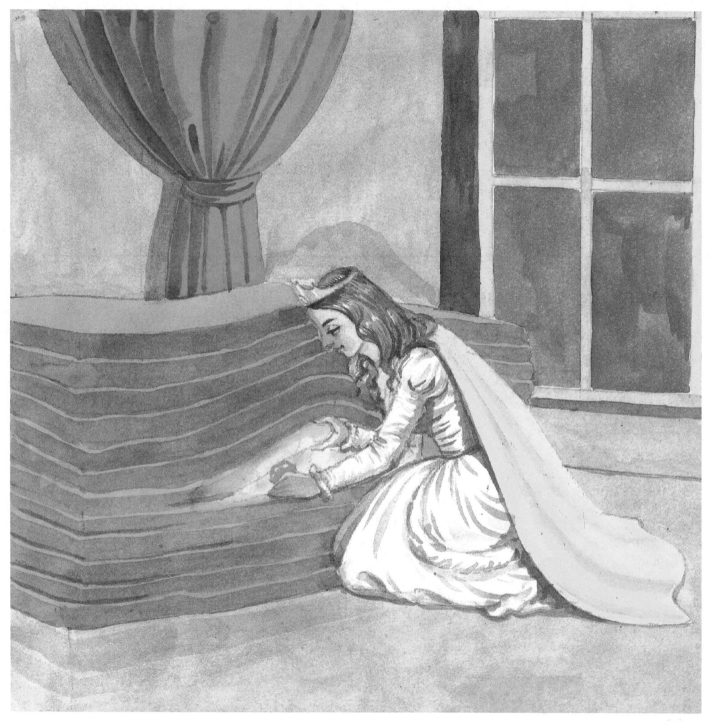

The Princess and the Ruby

As the night drew on, the little girl couldn't sleep. She only tossed and turned. A crack in the palace's guestroom provided ample room for icy wind to blow through. The little girl was also disturbed by some unknown kink in her bed.

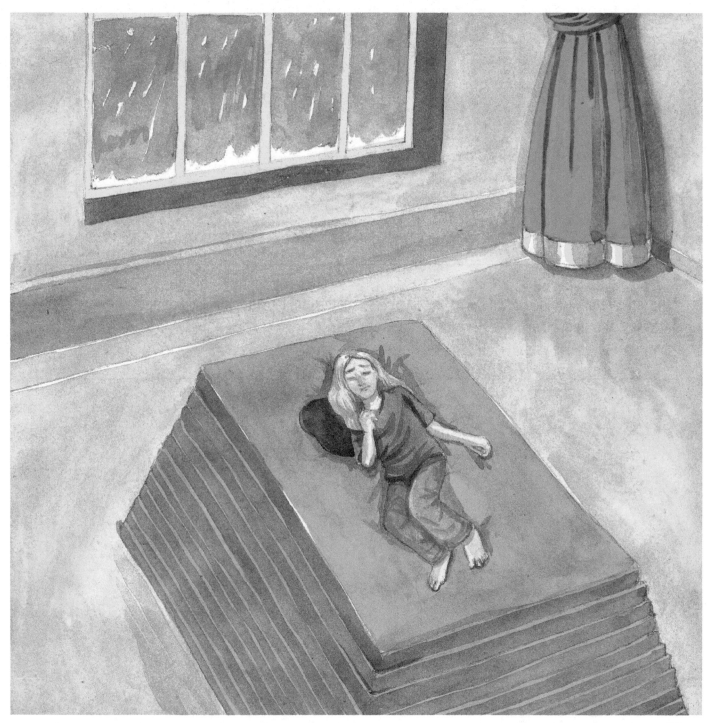

The Princess and the Ruby

The girl carefully climbed down the mountain of mattresses and stopped midway. Her eyes squinted at a shiny red object. She yanked it out. The girl walked to the problematic hole and promptly shoved the ruby into it.

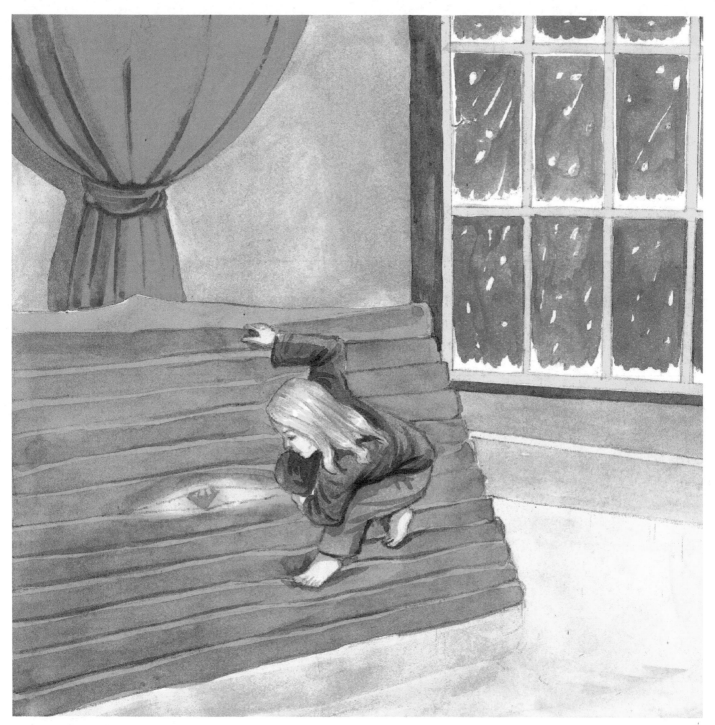

The Princess and the Ruby

Never one to complain, the little girl sat down on the bare carpet and let out a sigh of relief. Ever so carefully, she lined up her dear rocks in front of her.

She swayed gently back-and-forth until at long last she fell asleep.

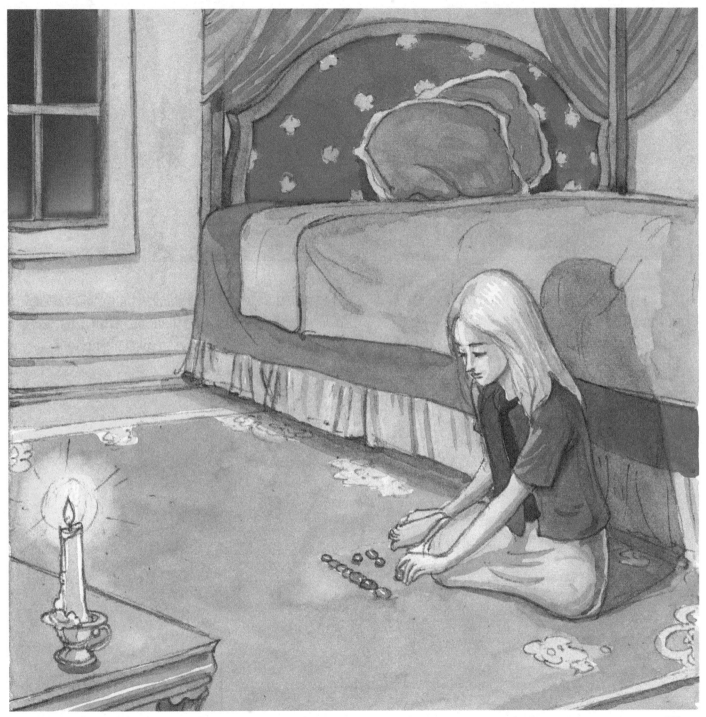

The Princess and the Ruby

"Did you manage to have a good night's rest?" the queen asked breathlessly.

The little girl didn't answer, but only continued to play with her rocks.

The new queen grinned. *I knew it! How could a child so different be one of us?* she thought. With utter satisfaction, she pranced over to collect her priceless ruby.

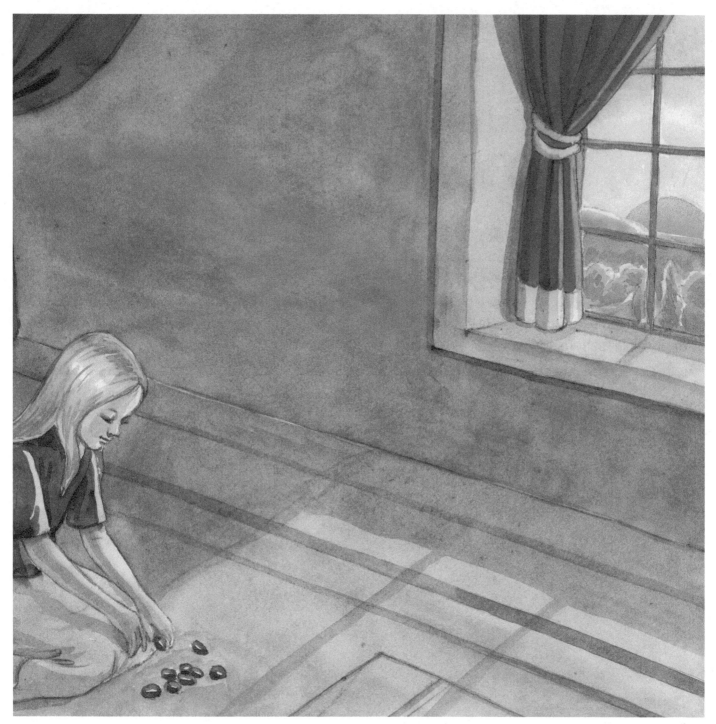

The Princess and the Ruby

The new queen stuck her hands into the center of the soft mattresses. Nothing was to be found. Again, the little girl spun around in circles.

As the girl spun, the new queen noticed the ruby shoved into the cracked window. She gasped in shock. "You *really* are the missing Princess!"

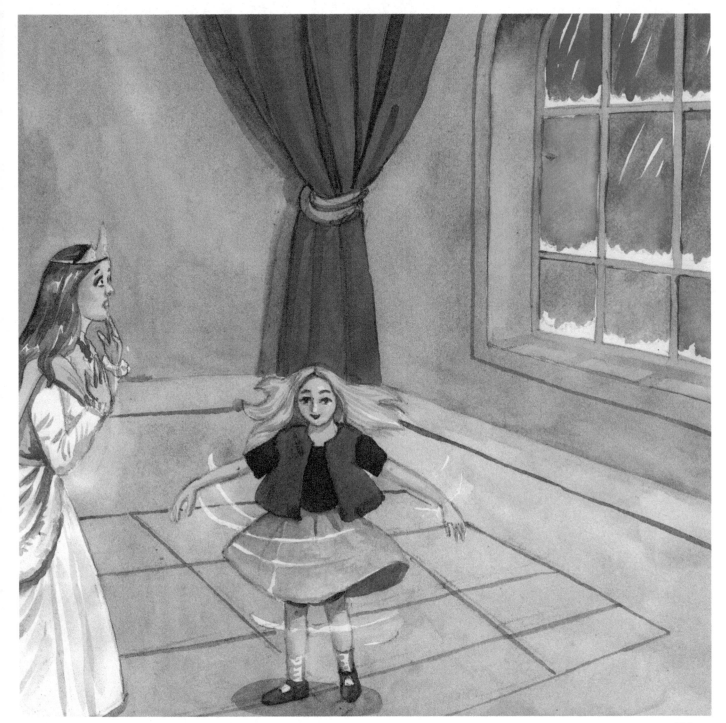

The Princess and the Ruby

With no expenses spared, a majestic party was held to celebrate the return of the missing princess. People travelled long distances to attend this one-of-a-kind kingdom event.

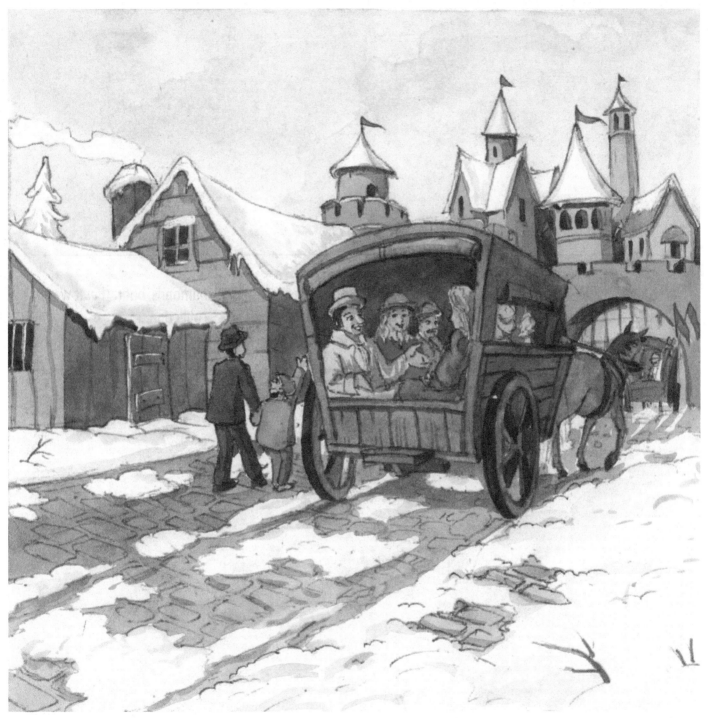

The Princess and the Ruby

The king and new queen hired only the best craftspeople to create a gold crown for their daughter. Like the little girl, it was unique. However, the crown did not bear traditional diamonds, but rather it was decorated with her rock collection.

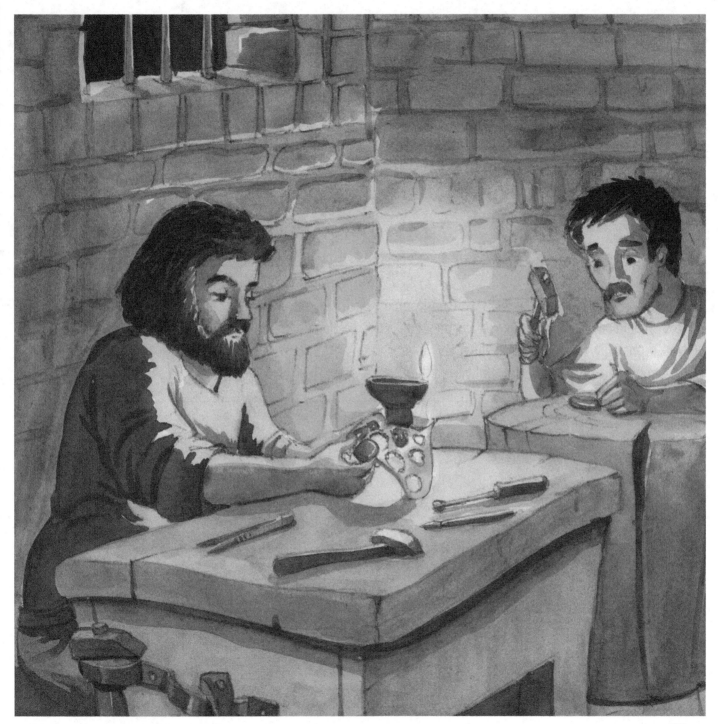

The Princess and the Ruby

To the princess' delight, the rocks were removable so she could line them up whenever she pleased. Not surprisingly, she had done so at her very own ceremony. The girl sat aside gracefully from the crowd, absorbed with her rock collection as the festivities went on.

THE END

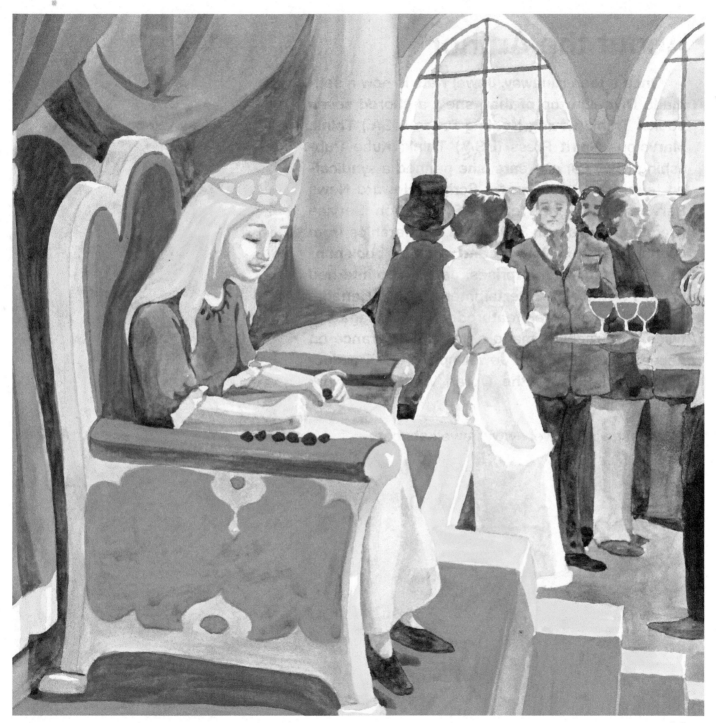

The Princess and the Ruby

About the Author

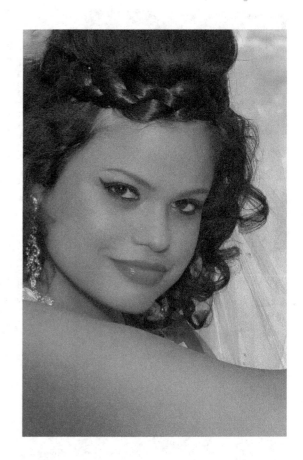

Once a teen runaway, Jewel Kats is now a self-made Diva. On top of that, she's authored seven books! Think: Loving Healing Press (USA.) Think: Marvelous Spirit Press (USA.) Think: Kube Publishing (UK.) For six years, she penned a syndicated teen advice column for Scripps Howard News Service (USA) and TorStar Syndication Service (Canada). She's won $20,000 in scholarships from Global Television Network and women's book publisher, Harlequin Enterprises. Jewel also interned in the TV studio of Entertainment Tonight Canada. Her books have been featured in Ability Magazine twice. She recently made a guest appearance on Accessibility in Action. Jewel appeared in a documentary series by the Oprah Winfrey Network (Canada) in 2012.

Please visit Jewel : www.jewelkats.com

Also by Jewel Kats

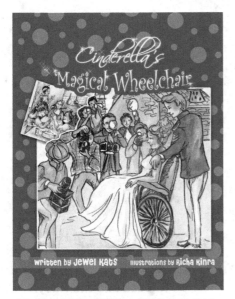

Cinderella's Magical Wheelchair:
An Empowering Fairy Tale

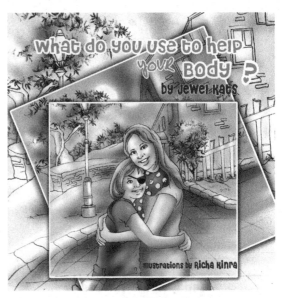

What Do You Use to Help Your Body?
Maggie Explores the World of Disabilities

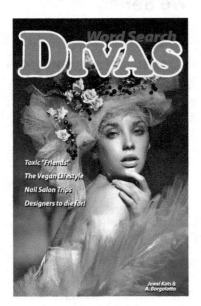

Word Search Divas

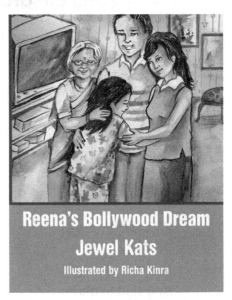

Reena's Bollywood Dream:
A Story about Sexual Abuse

www.JewelKats.com

Also by Jewel Kats

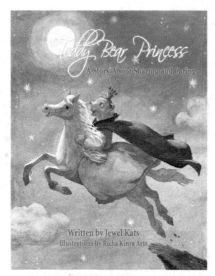

Teddy Bear Princess:
A Story about Sharing and Caring

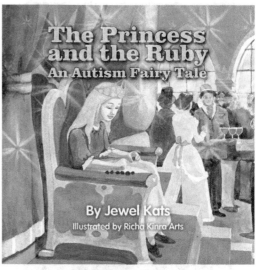

The Princess and the Ruby:
An Autism Fairy Tale

From the Growing with Love Series

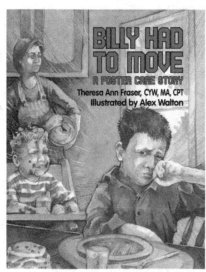

Billy Had to Move:
A Foster Care Story

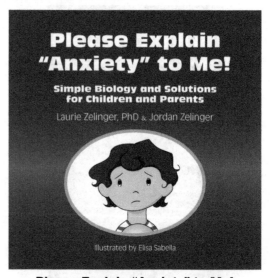

Please Explain "Anxiety" to Me!
Simple Biology & Solutiosn for Children

www.LHPress.com/growing-with-love

CPSIA information can be obtained at www.ICGtesting.com
Printed in the USA
LVOW02s0550090615

441719LV00011B/193/P

9 781615 991754